CULTURALLY ILL

CULTURALLY ILL

An Assessment of Healthcare by a VA Travel Nurse

Erin Elizabeth Paul, BSN, RN

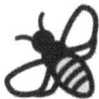

For correspondence, information, and permission requests, email Erin at book@hivehealthcoaching.com or send request to: PO Box 886 Moorhead, MN, 56561.

The content of this book is for general instruction only. Each person's physical, mental, emotional, and spiritual condition is unique. The instruction in this book is not intended to replace or interrupt the reader's relationship with a physician or other professional. Please consult your doctor for matters pertaining to your specific health and diet.

To connect with Erin and learn more about Hive Life Enhancement, visit hivehealthcoaching.com

ISBN-13: 978-0692534106
ISBN-10: 0692534105

Cover design: Alex Ehlen
Editor: Kirsten Lusty
Photo of Erin: Britta Trygstad

Printed in the United States of America

For the courageous visionaries of our time

Never believe that a few caring people can't change the world. For, indeed, that's all who ever have.

Margaret Mead

Contents

Acknowledgments

Without T, this book would not be what it is. *I've learned so much because of you.*

My parents have always supported me in all my ventures. *I love you, Mom. I love you, Dad.*

To my sister who is a nurse with a really big heart. *The world is better because of you, Sister.*

My brother's interest and involvement in this project was very meaningful. *Thank you, Brother.*

My grandfathers served our country in the armed services and then as farmers. *Forever in my heart..*

To my grandmothers who taught me about family, loyalty, and strength. *You are amazing women.*

This writing process was much more fun because of my animals. *Thanks for all the laughs, Kittos.*

To my best friend who has always believed in my dreams. *Dream big and believe, Bestie.*

My first Fargo friend has been very influential in my life. *It's a blessing to have met you, Trailblazer.*

To cross paths in Fargo with such a kindred spirit is thrilling. *Endless possibilities, Amethyst.*

Introduction

What our society accepts as *normal* in the
healthcare industry is disturbing and disgusting.

My purpose is to bring awareness to the signs and
symptoms of our culture's infection, its root cause,
and what we can do to stop this epidemic.

Stat.

Assessment

Healthcare

My first job in healthcare was at a local nursing home as a certified nursing assistant.

"All we ever do around here is eat," the lucid would say. It was true. Getting people out of bed, feeding them and laying them back down was about all I did on a shift. Up, down, up, down, up, down. The windows were never open. Days weren't spent outdoors. Many residents had no guests and others said family visited rarely. Residents had little interaction with anyone other than staff. There was no real human connection.

The place was lifeless.

The nurses spent their days handing out medications. I wondered how much more alive these frail humans would be if they were getting less drugs and more fresh air, sunshine, and love.

This surely did not inspire me to be a nurse.

Nursing was a good fit for my personality so I pursued the profession. I am very grateful for my education, degree and professional role, but I now wonder how much I was influenced by the job security of the profession.

Nurses are always in demand.

Nursing school had left me with the impression that career options as a new nurse were only the different units in a hospital. I was told I would eventually find my niche.

"Which one do you want to work in, Erin?"

None of them.

Hospital and hospitality are derived from the same Latin word, but hospitals are not hospitable. From the outside, they are massive structures and from the inside they are mind-boggling mazes. Florescent lights beam down in the cafeterias and "guest" rooms. Stale air lingers everywhere. Outside of their room windows, patients have brick walls to stare at while they lay in uncomfortable beds.

Sleep is a luxury during a hospital stay.

Professionals are always rushing from here to there, with little time to talk and less time to listen. Nurse stations are places to hear gossip about patients and coworkers. The hospital is not known for respectful relationships. During nursing orientation, nurses "eat their young" to establish dominance. Doctors are demeaning to nurses. Patients treat nurses as servants. And nursing assistants are dumped on by everyone. Literally.

Nothing about this environment suggests healing.

My first traumatic experience in the hospital as a professional was during nursing school. A morbidly obese senior woman lay there naked, legs spread wide and genitalia exposed. She had an eight-inch surgical incision along her groin. Her face was wrenched with pain and agony. The fresh surgical wound was open to air and on display for all to see.

Being a patient in the healthcare system is a very vulnerable position to be in. I have been there.

I was in my early twenties when I woke up with severe right-sided abdominal pain. I was a nurse at the time and figured it was my appendix. Even as a professional, this was a scary experience. When the emergency room doctor confirmed my diagnosis, he told me that my appendix would burst if I was not taken in for emergency surgery.

It didn't sound like I was being given an option.

Surgery was routine and without complications. I went home on oral pain pills with a bloated and tender tummy. When the pain meds wore off, I began reflecting on the whole situation.

When I went to the emergency room, I was scared and in severe pain. When the doctor told me what needed to be done, I did not question him.

From there, I was loaded up on a table where I was "put to sleep". Strangers then opened me up and removed a piece of my body. I knew this is what happened within the hospital walls but having actually gone through the experience, it was unsettling.

Was surgery really my only option?

The follow-up appointment made me feel even worse.

The surgeon took a mere two minutes to look at my incisions and that was that. There was no discussion about why my appendix became inflamed and what I should do to prevent further inflammation throughout the rest of my body.

I left the office confused and wondered why the professionals were not the least bit concerned about educating and empowering me.

A hospital stay is a prime opportunity to model healthful choices and behaviors. However, hospitals actually promote behaviors and provide the very choices that make people sick.

Most days at work, making time for lunch was difficult for me so I would raid the patients' pantry and fridge for snacks. Cheddar cheese with saltines and graham crackers with cream cheese were the norm. For a month, I was hooked on a popular "protein shake". My cravings would be so strong during my shift that I would sneak into the pantry and chug one.

This drink was turning into my drug so I looked into its ingredients. It contained *lots* of sugar and monosodium glutamate (MSG). MSG is a neurotoxic substance that causes us to eat or drink more. This was the same manufacturer of all the items in the vending machines. These machines were accessible to patients, visitors, and employees and were stocked with popular processed junk foods and sugary drinks.

How can people heal if they are being given highly processed, sugar-laden, food-like substances?

When I addressed these nutritional concerns with management, *customer satisfaction* was their primary concern. Apparently, if our "customers" didn't have a hamburger and fries on the menu they would go elsewhere for care. I was stunned. I thought our role in health care was to help people get well, not to facilitate the diet and lifestyle choices that led them to the hospital in the first place.

My first year as a nurse was disorienting. Into my second year, I was more confident in my position so I was able to process what I was actually doing. A twelve-hour shift consisted of me running from room to room, adjusting dangerous intravenous drugs, handing out pills, and administering IV pain meds every hour.

I was a drug-pusher.

Looking back on nursing school, I see how I was being prepped for this role.

My university was known for its prestigious nursing school. The school's 99% state board exam pass rate resulted in nursing courses that were brutal. I read textbook, after textbook, after textbook. There were many sleepless nights preparing my care plans, stressing over skills tests, memorizing classifications of drugs, and studying for difficult exams. Upon graduation, I was well prepared in knowing what could possibly go wrong with the body and what medication I'd be ordered to give when it does.

Over the years, the devastating effects of drug use have become very apparent to me. I'm not talking about illegal street drugs. I am talking about the drugs that are in typical homes across the United States-pharmaceutical drugs and prescription medications. I can easily count on one hand those I know whose life has been ruined or ended because of pharmaceutical drugs.

Prescription drugs now kill more people than illegal drugs.

Everybody is on drugs. New life is conceived of two persons on prescription medications. These children grow inside a womb of a woman taking drugs every day. Babies are born to mothers medicated with narcotics during labor. Children are being prescribed meds to calm them. Teenagers are taking pills for moods. Adults use medications for everything. Seniors plan their days according to their drug schedule.

Everybody is on drugs.

I remember going to the doctor's office regularly as a young child. I had chronic earaches. The doctor would quickly look into my ears, write a script for an antibiotic, and off we went to the pharmacy. Amoxicillin was a staple in my household. To this day I still remember its bubble gum flavor. There was never was a discussion about why I was having these ear infections and what could be done to prevent them.

In high school, I was having shortness of breath and nightly coughing fits. There was no question of what was causing these symptoms. I was not asked about my highly processed diet or my environment. My smoking habit was not discussed; instead, I was just told that I had asthma. The doctor prescribed me a once-a-day pill, a daily maintenance inhaler, and an inhaler for emergencies. The doctor said I would have to take these meds the rest of my life. I believed him.

We have been conditioned to think that we need medications to be well.

We are being hypnotized with drug commercials that flood the airwaves. The actors look healthy and happy. It's as if *that* is the magic pill that is going to make you feel good and be well. The images that you see are very different than what you are hearing from the seductive voice-over. The awful side effects are usually worse than the condition itself.

These mind-numbing advertisements are successfully convincing the general public that the solution to their health problems is a little white pill. The first drug is prescribed and then a second for the side effects of the first. Two becomes three and on it goes.

"Ask you doctor today if this pill is right for you."

My last day as a hospital floor nurse is a day I will always remember. I stood before a man with kidney disease and handed him two medicine cups full of pills. Kidneys filter the waste out of the blood. Giving a man a mouthful of meds for his already exhausted kidneys to filter is not logical.

This just doesn't feel right.

I made a commitment to myself that day to be a drugless practitioner.

Diet and lifestyle choices have a huge impact on our health so how is prescribing and administering drugs really helping people get well?

During my first year as a nurse, my stress levels were off the charts. I was working twelve-hour night shifts; I'd toss and turn all day long when I should have been sleeping. On my days off, I would use alcohol to come down from the work week.

When I planned a roadtrip with my girlfriends, I was ready to let all my anxieties go and have a great vacation. At the time, the only way I knew how to do this was with alcohol. We stayed up all night drinking into the early morning and I was running on adrenaline throughout the rest of the day. By the end of the week, I'd slept no more hours than the equivalent of two full nights of rest.

When you don't sleep, real life can quickly turn into a bizarre dream. I was having grandiose thoughts, severe paranoia, and acting irrationally. Not knowing what was happening, my friends took me to the hospital. I have vivid memories from the emergency room, but remember nothing after they put in an IV and administered a sedative. I woke up that evening in a padded room in the psych ward. After a nice long rest and a warm bowl of soup, I was beginning to feel like myself again.

There was no privacy and I was not given the option to make any decisions. Only one nurse acknowledged and interacted with me as a fellow human being. It was as if the other nurses thought they were superior to me. Or perhaps they were afraid of me. It was difficult to be stripped of my personal dignity, but to have professionals who did not treat me with respect was worse.

That day I learned the importance of nurses being accepting, kind-hearted, and hospitable.

When it came time for med pass, I was not given the choice to take the drug I'd been prescribed. I was told I had to follow doctor's orders, but they hadn't even met with me since I woke from the sedation I received in the emergency room.

This was an outrage.

The next day, I sat at a long table before six different professionals. They informed me my drug screen was negative. When I asked why I had had these experiences, electrolyte imbalances and sleep deprivation were briefly mentioned. Although it was obvious to me that my extreme party week was the main cause, this was not really discussed by the professionals. When I told them I was back to my normal self and ready to go home, they trumped my request and told me they were going to keep me for another night.

The following day I was sent home with a prescription for an antipsychotic and a diagnosis of a bi-polar episode. I don't recall why I filled that script, but I did. I took those pills for three days and lived in an emotionless fog.

No thanks, Doc.

Six months later, I applied for a new health care plan for basic coverage. When my premiums were $200 more every month than my previous comparable plan, I asked the insurance company why. They had on record that I filled a prescription for an antipsychotic. It was the medication that I should never have been prescribed in the first place.

The VA Way

The realities about healthcare were becoming more evident and I was feeling burnt out. When I discovered travel nursing, I knew this was a much better fit. My assignments would be anywhere from three to six months, so I would have the opportunity to see the country.

When I saw a rare commercial for the Veterans Health Administration on late night television, I figured this was a sign. Though I knew little about the VA, I applied to their traveling nurse program.

My first impression of the VA could have been better but it was accurate.

They lost my application, which had taken hours to complete. Then, they asked that I send it again via postal service. Next, they misplaced my references. After resubmitting the requested documents, I was informed that my paperwork had been buried on someone's desk all along.

So...apparently you all aren't very organized.

In the private sector, travel agencies can have nurses on assignment in a few weeks, so I was not expecting such a long process from the VA. The hire process took three entire months. My contact in Human Resources even said this was twice as fast as she'd seen any VA travel nurse be hired on. I imagine my application was expedited so they'd stop receiving my Friday "just following up" calls.

It was finally official, though. I would be touring the United States as a VA travel nurse.

It wasn't long thereafter I started feeling mistreated.

The VA did not provide any paid time for orienting myself to my temporary new life. I was expected to show up to my new duty station on Sunday and begin work on Monday. "The budget" did not allow reimbursement for time spent securing comfortable housing, organizing healthy meals and navigating safely to work. This would all be paid out of my pocket.

One manager confessed his facility used VA travel nurses because they were cheaper than permanent staff. Travelers were paid the same as permanent staff, but were not given vacation days, sick leave and, until recently, federal employee health benefits.

I'm going to repeat that.

I was a registered nurse for the Veterans Health Administration and I was *not* given the option for health benefits.

I received a daily per diem for meals and incidentals, so this offset what the VA was not affording me. However, shortly after I began, a large percentage of this was no longer reimbursed. This ended up being around a two thousand dollar pay cut in a three-month period.

In facility after facility, I witnessed the waste of government funds.

Employees would shamelessly admit that they hadn't done anything all day. They would joke about starting the weekend early. People would gather by the coffee pot for an hour in the morning talking about weekend fun with family. The fifteen minute mandated break would turn into thirty. Then, being caught up in the latest VA gossip, a thirty minute lunch would turn into an hour. Throughout the day there were interruptions by coworkers who were away from their desk, not working. Ample time was spent on unimportant emails, unproductive meetings and pointless education. Twenty minutes at the end of the day was spent talking about evening plans unless the employee had already left early.

And the government is cutting my pay?!

As a traveler, I had to be very organized. Many times I felt like I was the only one who had any organizational skills whatsoever. Even after hours of traveling on the road the day prior, I was typically less disoriented than the Human Resources department. "Ah?! Who are you again? They told me you weren't coming for another week. Why did they tell you to come here? You aren't supposed to come to this office first. Go there and then come back!"

At one facility, my first two hours on the job were spent listening to my point-of-contact grumble about my arrival. She didn't have my file complete and didn't "have time for all this". As quickly as she could, this woman took me to my new department. The nurse in the department was surprised about my arrival. She said she hadn't expected me for a week, but began sharing her daily routine.

"This is nothing like the job they offered me during my phone interview," I said. I wouldn't have been surprised if I was interviewed for the wrong position because disorganization is the norm but I inquired further.

My point-of-contact mixed me up with another nurse and had taken me to the wrong department.

I always arrived to my new assignment with a smile on my face and enthusiastic to work. My smile quickly faded as time and time again I faced rude, incompetent, and sluggish employees. All too often, my arrival and presence seemed like an inconvenience.

After nineteen hours on the road, I received an email at 1530 stating I was not to report the following day. I inquired about the delay promptly and was told I hadn't been cleared for work. I asked for clarification and it was revealed that one person in their Human Resources "needed to hit enter".

"We sent him an email but haven't heard back."

Perhaps you could you call and speak to someone directly?

Many conversations in the VA happen via email when a verbal dialogue would be more appropriate. Perhaps email is primarily used to create a trail of accountability, but I found that in using email, even with the utmost clarity, matters were not fully addressed and sometimes not even acknowledged.

Maybe email is overused because calling on the telephone is also ineffective. Employees screen their calls or aren't ever at their desks. Response to voicemails is not prompt, if at all.

Rarely would I receive confirmation of emails or voicemails. "Got your message. Working on it. Will get back to you within 48 hours." Simple communication such as this does not happen. Often I was left not knowing whether my message was received or if anyone was doing anything about it.

More times than not, I was encouraged to send an email. I was warned that any other type of communication would "just slow them down even more." Email has its benefits, but it is not always the best means of communication. More often, I preferred a verbal dialogue where I could have a conversation and not have to wait for opens, forwards, and replies.

How can the VA provide "excellence in care" to Veterans if disorganization and miscommunication is the norm?

When I was direct in asking people to do their job, I was met with hostility and a defensive attitude. I never understood why it was so offensive to ask someone to do their job. It is their job, right?!

Employees always have to follow up with coworkers to ensure matters are addressed and resolved for Veterans. It is *really* frustrating to always be asking for something that should have already been done.

My first assignment was in a small side unit working with a night nurse who was awful, unkind, and lazy. This woman was the unit bully. She spent her night paying bills and Facebooking. Typically, I kept my distance. However, one night, I requested her assistance to turn a morbidly obese Veteran in bed. She told me I should let him sleep. I was aware of the importance of sleep but I also knew the deadly potential of a bed sore. I shared my rationale for my plan of care and yet she still refused to help me. When I reminded her of how important it was for us to work together, she pulled me out of our unit.

We were in front of the main nurses station where she began yelling at me. Her claims were all attacks on my personality and were very belittling. I stood tall. When she finally finished her tantrum, I told her all I was asking for was assistance with a Veteran in need, which was her job. The scuffle was the talk of the day shift and when I returned that evening, one nurse even thanked me. "I've been wanting to tell her that for ten years," she confessed.

Ten years? What a miserable work environment!

As a traveling nurse, I never expected much training when I arrived at my assignment. Travelers are expected to hit the ground running. Typical orientation was "here is the break room, that is the med cart, here is the supply closet, and this is our daily routine." I grew accustomed to identifying resourceful staff and asking lots of questions. There were few expectations of me as a travel nurse. As long as I kept my Veterans safe and didn't kill anyone, I had done my job.

I assumed that I received expedited training because I was a traveling nurse. This was not the case.

When I had the opportunity to work in a growing department, I witnessed the orientation process for new employees in my same position.

The disorganization and inadequate training for new staff was baffling. These employees were later reprimanded and ridiculed for not performing well in their position.

I couldn't understand why new employees were not receiving thorough training.

At one point, I shared some helpful tips with a new coworker. Her preceptor, a seasoned VA nurse said, "You are giving away all my secrets. Now, she is going to have a leg up on me."

Is this a competition?

At a different facility, I needed a mobile phone for my position as a visiting nurse. Management could easily have completed most of the paperwork prior to my arrival; instead, I had to run this and that, here and there, for him and her. When I put the pressure on employees who were "necessary" in the lengthy process, it was as if I was being impatient.

My assignment was only for three months and it took almost a month to get my work phone.

This should not be so difficult.

In the most dysfunctional facility I experienced, my work-space was in a large, cluttered storage room. I was given a portable computer and my seating was a transportation cot. The lack of preparedness with my arrival was nothing new so I was somewhat patient, but I soon realized that my situation was not going to change.

Across the hall was an office with two work spaces, one that I have never seen occupied. When I inquired with the woman in the office, she was very matter-of-fact in that saying the computer was for the social workers. I inquired further and she admitted it was only used occasionally for social work students and interns.

On this particular day, my computer was nowhere to be found and the cot was snatched out from under me for an emergency transport. After an hour of unsuccessfully assembling a work-space, I moved to the open computer designated for social workers.

My new office-mate was not the least bit welcoming.

When I stepped out of the office, she left for a meeting in the conference room right next door and locked me out. She was the only person with a key to the door so in order to continue working, I had her pulled from her meeting to let me in. She rolled her eyes in front of the whole group and stomped out.

"I knew this was going to happen," she exclaimed.

This work environment was unacceptable and no longer was I going to compete for work-space just so I could do my job. This was the same facility that it took me a month to get a work phone. All I was asking for was a professional work area so I could perform basic tasks necessary in my current role to serve Veterans. When I addressed this matter with my manager, she responded, "Let me make some calls." An hour later, I was in an office space that was designated for the previous nurse in my position and had been empty all along.

How can the VA be successful in delivering care to Veterans if employees are not given proper training and the necessary tools to do their job well?

Fresh out of the service and motivated to work with other Vets, a combat Veteran was hired at the VA. His office space doubled as the supply room that contained the fax machine, printer, coffee pot, and employee mail boxes. This small space was a revolving door of employees, interruptions and distractions. A work environment such as this, would be stressful for anyone. For a combat Vet who was trained to be aware of his surroundings at all times, this was incredibly stressful and over-stimulating.

These matters were brought to the attention of his manager numerous times. As a much better suited office nearby was underutilized, this Veteran employee remained in the terrible space for years.

If Veteran employees are treated so poorly, why would Veteran patients be treated any differently?

To remain in the VA system, Veterans must be seen for a yearly check-up. I've met many younger Veterans who dread going to the VA, even just once a year. It's no wonder why. They face the same disrespect and rudeness that I experienced as an employee. VA employees make Veterans feel like an inconvenience when the employees have to do their job. Unsolicited, timely, and thorough assistance is the exception rather than the norm as it should be. When Veterans lose patience with the unapologetic cultural norms and express this frustration, they are considered hostile.

This is the experience of a relatively healthy Veteran receiving little care from the VA.

The Veterans Administration is a significant stressor in the lives of Veterans. Getting a piece of mail from the VA creates anxiety for many.

It is a struggle for Veterans to get service-related injuries recognized. The medical model doesn't recognize the body as a whole system so certain health issues are often considered "unrelated" to their time in the service. Some surrender after years of one denied claim after another.

When I started working with Veterans, I recognized the complexity of their health compared to civilians. Veterans also tolerate what most civilians would never survive. As a result of this, the horrors of healthcare are magnified.

I was caring for a Veteran post-op who had been diagnosed with throat cancer. The doctors had removed a third of his jaw and the rest of the area was blasted with radiation. There were severe burns and his pain was uncontrollable. He said, "They didn't tell me it was going to be like this."

Many VA facilities are teaching hospitals so I witnessed new interns excited with any unique experience. I imagined this man's team of doctors more concerned with a learning opportunity than his quality of life. I wondered how many details were left out or were not emphasized to ensure this Vet would continue with that plan of care.

Another Veteran I was caring for had spent weeks in the hospital. He was dying a slow and painful death. This Vet was incredibly confused as a result of liver failure. He also had not slept in days. Whether or not it was a moment of lucidity, this man clearly stated that he just wanted to go home to die.

They told him he couldn't leave.

If a person wishes to die at home, shouldn't that person have the right to do so?

This is all so wrong.

I was working with a Veteran who had diabetes and was experiencing high blood sugars. My role as a nurse and coach is to teach people about the addictiveness of sugar and support them to get off of this serious drug. When this happens, they can quit destroying their bodies with sugar.

The Veteran and I talked about diabetes in the simplest terms. I discovered that he didn't know that sugar was in most foods. He was interested in learning the different names of sugar so he could identify it in the ingredient list of foods he typically ate. He was encouraged to replace these with healthier options.

This type of list could easily be found on the internet, but I had been instructed to provide only "approved" education to Veterans. I contacted the nutrition department to see what they had available. The dietician said they had nothing of the sort.

I shared this Veteran's interest in learning more about sugar. She responded sharply, "Just put in a diabetes education consult." The Veteran already had a consultation with the dietician and said it was not helpful. This was the same thing I had heard from countless others.

When I told her I was concerned this Veteran didn't know how to identify sugar in the ingredient list, her response was ridiculous. "We don't teach them that and you and I can't be teaching them different things. We only teach them how to read the daily values and we have been doing it like that for thirty years. Just put in a consult."

Just because something has been done for thirty years, does not mean we need to keep doing it.

Progressive medical doctors are managing diabetes with a plant-based diet combined with daily movement and self-love. This approach is much simplier and sometimes diabetes is even reversed.

With the outdated approach, managing diabetes is often a significant life stressor. Veterans are taught how to "control" their blood sugars. Their days are filled with pricking their finger tips, counting carbs, and self-injecting insulin. Many check their blood sugar four times a day and take insulin each time. Some Veterans become obsessed with levels being "within normal limits" but yet continue eating a diet full of sugar. The only thing that changes is the amount of insulin they take.

Insulin is a very dangerous drug and a simple mistake can lead to death. The deadly potential is not emphasized by professionals or respected by many of those with use insulin.

Despite advances in diabetes care, the VA maintains an outdated approach to managing diabetes. The VA continues providing Veterans with one-time use needles, expensive testing strips, a deadly drug, and a plan that is not addressing the real problem, a poor diet and lifestyle. This plan does not improve Veterans' quality of life and only encourages the dependency on yet another substance, sugar *and* insulin.

Some Veterans had mental health and drug abuse issues before serving in the military. They now use the VA to supply the pharmaceutical drugs that they are abusing. Combat service is just an excuse to continue the substance abuse.

One Veteran's ex-spouse admits, "He would experiment with drugs on the street to find what high he liked best and then go to the VA for a prescription. He knew exactly what to tell the doctors to get which drugs he wanted."

This Vet would rationalize his addiction, "Why would the VA prescribe it to me if I didn't need it?"

The available treatment options for Veterans are not always effective. A majority of post-911 Veterans I have met have a strong desire to explore complementary modalities. These are alternatives to the current allopathic approach that is seen throughout the healthcare system. Like everything in the VA, providing access to these different modalities is limited by policy, procedure, and protocol.

The VA utilizes the scientific "evidence-based"

approach. Unfortunately, profit and politics are a driving force for the necessary research for evidence-based practices. As a result, modalities like shamanism, herbalism and energy healing are not recognized as treatment options.

If Veterans and outside practitioners are finding success in modalities, why are Veterans not presented with these options? What better evidence is needed than Veterans saying, "This is working!"?

Pharmaceutical drug use is the typical treatment for our Veterans. Whether or not they desire to use these drugs, their symptoms are being masked and they remain ill. This is not serving our Veterans. While the VA slowly broadens its acceptable practices and prescription drug use continues, twenty-two Veterans kill themselves everyday.

This is unacceptable.

I had the opportunity to work in one of the newest VA programs where I did home visits and provided support to caregivers of post-911 Veterans. This program had so much potential to provide health coaching services to families in need. Instead, most of the time was spent doing paperwork and creating more stress in Veterans lives with intrusive home visits.

Within weeks, among the many issues I recognized was poor resource utilization. If my position was stationed at a different VA facility an hour away, my drive time would be cut in half and I would have more time to reach Veterans and their loved ones.

This was addressed with the nurse manager. She disregarded the information and said to me, "I just oversee this program for the social workers. I don't want to step on anyone's toes."

Dominance over the care of Veterans is an issue throughout the VA system. Professionals and departments are territorial over aspects of care and the VA itself does not do well collaborating with outside assistance. A colleague of mine witnessed a manager throwing away resources that were provided from an outside facility wanting to support Veterans.

When I told my manager I had become a certified health coach, I thought she would be interested in how I could use these skills to better serve Veterans. She said, instead, "Know that you cannot work with Veterans in private if you are employed by the VA. There is a conflict of interest."

When the "VA scandal" hit the news, the nation was talking about the failures of the system. There was a national outcry for accountability, leadership and change. I was receiving emails everyday full of bureaucratic talk about culture change and the ICARE philosophy: integrity, commitment, advocacy, respect and excellence. Assuming the VA would be looking for new leaders, I was driven to create a wellness program for post-911 Veterans.

My vision began with the house on the premises that was being used for a workout area exclusively for employees. My plan was to transform this house into a hospitable home-like space for Veterans including a kitchen for cooking demonstrations, a meditation room, and a library full of useful resources.

The environment would be peaceful and calm.

Veterans would be at the center of this program. They would have a voice in determining what modalities were offered. They would be engaged in creating the community that so many of them long for and need.

After boldly presenting this plan to top management, they showed no interest in my enthusiasm, my energy, or my ideas. I was prodded along like most forward-thinking, motivated professionals in the VA.

We need to be doing so much more for Veterans.

I returned to my department where we had a meeting to discuss "numbers". This program had grown so rapidly that we were unable to meet documentation requirements set by the national

VA. For every Veteran enrolled, the documentation was taking four hours, which was excessive. No one was using the information that we collected and we all agreed the paperwork did not improve the quality of care. The more time we spent catching up on charting, the less time we were providing the monitoring our program had promised.

When the manager clearly stated documentation was the priority, I was disheartened. I shared what was most important to the discussion, "These aren't *numbers*. These are *people*. All these *numbers* you are talking about are *Veterans*."

My obvious statement didn't change her decision. After the meeting this manager came to me personally. She said, as if she'd convince me otherwise, "I know this doesn't seem right, Erin, but it's the way it has to be done."

It doesn't have to be like this, nor should it be.

Diagnosis

I worked in six different VA medical centers throughout the United States and have witnessed the depth of this toxic culture. Clever acronyms and shallow efforts are not going to change the VA.

The failure to cooperate and collaborate exists among employees, Veterans, programs, departments, VA facilities, and outside resources. Disorganization, power struggles, and impaired communication throughout the system are all having a negative impact on the employees providing care, and, most importantly, on the Veterans.

New employees are given nothing more than what is required for their job and sometimes not even that. It's an *exception*, rather than the norm, for personnel to complete their duties in a timely and effective manner without being asked.

Holding others accountable is difficult in a culture where unaccountability is acceptable. Those who speak up often experience ridicule and retaliation. People in leadership positions are not good leaders; they are more concerned with maintaining status quo than raising the standards. The personnel and policy makers at the top are far removed from Veterans and their needs.

There are long chains of command and lots of red

tape that delays care for Veterans. Dispersing new health information takes considerable amounts of time and proposing new ideas and initiating change is met with great resistance. When change needs to happen, it must go through many already slow-moving channels. There are limitations in providing only "evidence-based" approaches.

These politics are preventing improvement in the quality of care delivered and prevent Veterans from receiving comprehensive and progressive care.

Many employees are oblivious to how their destructive behaviors are contributing to the systemic infection. There is a lack of awareness of whose time and money is wasted. Employees do not realize the negative impact of this attitude on the system. Well-intending, dedicated, and hard-working employees often succumb to the system and grow more complacent everyday. Some are hiding out until retirement, chained to the golden handcuffs of the VA, while others resign and more than a few Vets have said, "it's all the good ones that leave."

The failure of the Veterans Health Administration is not solely due to the toxic environment.

Healthcare professionals are not taught how to practice and promote wellness or help people be well. Instead of addressing the root cause of health issues, drugs are prescribed and surgery is scheduled. This encourages people to ignore the important messages from the body and is preventing the opportunity to truly heal. The result is a worsening of the condition and more health complications.

We are not taught how to understand the body and the doctors are now the ones who have authority over it. They are the only ones who can translate its messages. Unfortunately, they speak in a language of only pills and procedures.

Healthcare is based on a Western medical model that separates us into body systems. We are not seen as whole beings. For every area of the body, there is a specialist. A person may have several issues that are all related to one another but because they are in different systems, the connection is lost.

A majority of illness and disease today is caused by everyday choices. This fact is being overlooked.

People live solely on food-like substances and abuse socially acceptable drugs like caffeine. There are high levels of stress, excessive amounts of working, loveless relationships and a lack of daily movement. People and professionals fail to see the link between diet and lifestyle and energy, infertility, lack of sex drive, anxiety, fluctuating moods, and general unhappiness.

It is only the physical and mental symptoms that are addressed in the healthcare system. This a major reason why Western medicine and the VA are failing our Veterans. The physical wounds from war are obvious, but emotional and spiritual wounds are unseen. These deep wounds are rarely tended to.

Our emotional and spiritual health are not recognized much in society, either. We are not taught to explore, relate to and care for these deeper dimensions of ourselves.

We are not taught to trust in ourselves. But we *are* taught trust in our doctors.

A man once told me that he was putting his life in his doctor's hands. He was dead a week later.

People put all of their faith in the healthcare system. They believe their doctors will *save* them and *fix* any health issues that occur. In believing so, they give their power away. They give their power to a system driven by scandalous insurance and self-interested pharmaceutical companies.

This is why the current healthcare system is less *health*-care than it is *sick*-care. The best customers are the sick ones that keep coming back. Healthy people just aren't good for business.

Healthcare is just another industry more concerned with profit than people.

Cannabis is a substance that many Veterans prefer over pharmaceutical drugs to manage symptoms of PTSD. They report that this herb is more effective and has significantly milder side effects compared to prescription medications.

Cannabis has been around for thousands of years and sacred in some cultures, but there are lies being told about this herb to The People and the media twists the debate into a public health concern. If the government was truly concerned about public health, sugar and prescription drugs are far more important conversations.

Cannabis remains illegal because it's a threat to pharmaceutical profit, not because it's a threat to The People.

It's all about the money.

In our country, youngsters are persuaded with money and educational opportunities to join the military. Many are living a family legacy of serving our country. For some, the military is one of their few options out of poverty, while others are longing for and honored to be part of something much bigger than themselves.

These young men and women are plucked right out of high school. They are broken down, rebuilt into machines, and sent off to fight corporate wars in the name of freedom.

When service members are no longer valuable to the warmongers, they are discarded.

Veterans are labeled as disabled, disgruntled, and diseased. They are feared and portrayed as crazy. They are told they will have to live with PTSD the rest of their lives.

There are lengthy trials of pharmaceutical drugs that have serious side effects, which sometimes lead to death.

All of these drugs are like Band-Aids on deep, bleeding wounds that were not tended to when these men and women returned from war.

Veterans have seen their country from a much different perspective.

Their very survival was dependent on their ability to be a unit. Communication, cooperation, and teamwork is what kept these men and women alive overseas, but they return to their country where there is no accountability, all channels of communication are impaired, and there is very little togetherness.

Many Veterans no longer feel right living the life they once lived. Some choose a life of solitude or homelessness after rejecting our society. Others dream of running away from it all.

It's no wonder Vets have "difficulty reintegrating into civilian life." Society is sick.

The most important civil duty is to be a consumer. Next, the most important is to keep your lawn green and groomed. Holidays are celebrated with sales and shopping events.

The newest technology, the trendiest clothes, and the most expensive cars will earn you status. At a very young age, we learn how to be competitive and are taught that being on top is what matters.

Money is worshipped and success is valued above all. People strive to acquire wealth, social status, and material possessions, believing this is the path to true happiness.

When people are most concerned with profit and power, they are sick. Whatever it may be, land, money, or materials, the need to acquire more and more is an addiction. This illness has been long ignored and actually rewarded in society.

This is an epidemic.

Those sick with greed are ruining our school systems, government agencies, businesses, religious organizations, and military, among many, many others. We now live in a country where ruthless exploitation, profiteering of others' problems, and creation of problems for profit is socially acceptable.

This socially encouraged addiction is an infection resulting in the destruction of *everything*.

Brand new mothers receive little, if any, paid time off and are financially forced back to work. Parents can't afford not to work so children are raised by strangers in day care. School-aged children are taught how to conform and obey. Teenagers are told through manipulative marketing what they "need" to be beautiful during their emotionally delicate years. End-of-life decisions for the elderly are less about dignity than they are about the dollar.

Mother Earth is being stripped of her finite resources. Farmland is being poisoned with chemicals, waterways are being polluted and trees and ancient rainforests are being bulldozed for cattle grazing and oil drilling.

Animals are being factory farmed and living in horrendous conditions. They are confined, raped, kidnapped, neglected, abused, and then murdered.

When we experience symptoms, illness, and disease, our bodies are telling us something in our life is out of balance. These are messages.

The ills throughout our culture tell us the same.

Increasing natural disasters, growing childhood poverty, and constant war are very loud messages to get our attention.

Our current way of living is out of balance and unsustainable.

Humans are actually merciful, compassionate, and kind. Witness human behavior in the aftermath of a natural disaster. People take care of one another and they are altruistic, putting the wellbeing of others before their own. They come together to solve problems. There is camaraderie and social solidarity. There is an outpouring of love, generosity, and acts of kindness.

This is the *true* nature of humanity.

In a society where money is valued over life, people are acting less human than ever.

Diagnosis: spiritual distress.

<u>Goals</u>

- *Know Your Self*
- *Own Your Power*

You are a powerful being.

Think of Anne Frank, Mother Teresa, and Florence Nightingale. These are just a few examples of everyday people that had a significant impact on the world.

One person does make a difference.

In a world of religious dogma and indoctrination, we do not learn how powerful we truly are as individuals. We are not taught to look inward and develop a relationship with our spiritual self.

Instead, we are told to put blind faith in politicians, prophets and providers.

Establishing a trusting relationship with your spirit self is empowering. This wise, inner being delivers dependable guidance and provides endless, loving support. For when you can trust yourself first and foremost, others are unable to lead you astray.

Confidence and self-esteem emerge as this

relationship with your spiritual self is strengthened. You are able to see your life purpose with more clarity. You are able to trust that you are fully supported to bring your gifts to the world.

As more people look inward for answers, express their divine self and live their truth, the world is that much closer to peace and harmony.

Looking inward may be intimidating.
Acknowledging your power may be terrifying.
Own it and you'll see how truly powerful you are.

You are more in control of your life than what you have been told.

It's time to take your power back.

Recommendations

There are six steps you can take to develop a more intimate relationship with yourself and realize your power.

Start spending more time with yourself and less time in relationships that are unfulfilling. Making quality time for *you* is a great way to start having a stronger connection with your spiritual self. Cherish this time and release any guilt about tending to your personal needs.

Your spiritual self speaks in whispers and is easy to disregard, especially if you have never been taught to listen. This is similar to someone trying to talk to you when the music is really loud. It's difficult to hear them. Perhaps you don't even know they are talking to you. To have a decent conversation, your must turn down the music.

This is similar to the mind.

When you quiet the chattering mind and tune out the distractions of society, communicating with your spiritual self becomes much easier.

Incorporate these practices into your every day life and you can experience subtle shifts and significant changes in all aspects of your life.

Step One: Breathe

Breathing is very important; humans can survive only minutes without oxygen, but at a young age, incorrect techniques are learned and little attention is given to breathing from there on. Shallow breathing exacerbates pain and contributes to various health issues, such as anxiety.

Watch a baby breathe and you will see baby's belly rise. This is called diaphragmatic breathing and is the correct breathing technique.

Observe your breathing.

Does your chest puff out? Do your shoulders rise? If so, you are not allowing the complete expansion of your lungs, which is necessary for your body and brain to get optimal levels of oxygen.

Raise your arms above your head and breathe. Notice how your abdomen extends? In this position, you automatically breathe correctly. Expanding your belly when you breathe may feel awkward at first, but eventually it will feel more natural.

Upon waking, begin your day with at least six deep breaths. Breathe in the freshness of the new day. Exhale and let go of any worries. A simple mantra like "breathe in, breathe out" or "peace, calm" is helpful in taking your awareness from your thoughts and bringing it to your breathing.

End your day with a minute of breathing as well. Inhale and welcome the stillness of the night. Exhale and release any tension from the day.

Incorporating conscious breathing into your day can relieve anxiety, decrease stress, and boost energy. Post reminders in areas you frequent to prompt you throughout the day to consciously breathe.

Just breathe.

Step Two: Slow Down

Our way of life has become so fast paced. People are living in a constant state of anxiety and don't even know it. This has become their normal way of living.

There is no time to breathe. Perhaps this is why people in our society are so anxious.

Taking time to consciously breathe will help you slow it down. Being aware of your breathing will bring you into the moment and impact the way you experience time.

When did you last pause to take in the life that surrounds you?

Any moment is an opportunity to reconnect with your breathing and slow down.

Take a moment before eating and connect with your breath. Express gratitude for your meal, smell your food, and notice your taste buds. Enjoy your food as you taste, chew, and swallow. Be present.

Mealtimes will be more relaxed and eating slower allows the body time to properly digest foods.

This mindfulness practice is great for shower time and especially during sex.

Paying attention to the moon cycle and living

accordingly can drastically change the way you experience time. Many people are familiar with the sun's routine, rise and fall. How familiar are you with the moon cycle?

When the moon is new, she is positioned between the sun and Earth where she is unseen by those on Earth. Each day the moon rises about an hour later.

A few days past the new moon, look near the sun at sunset and there you will see the moon's crescent. For the next few weeks, watch her wax across the night sky until she rises full. The full moon rises as the sun sets and over the next few weeks, the moon will wane across the day sky, appearing smaller until she is dark once again.

The moon has an influence on energy levels, natural body cycles, moods, and even the progression of projects. Following the moon cycle can bring more balance and harmony into your life.

Life doesn't just rise and fall. Life waxes and wanes.

Step Three: Be Still

Meditation is the practice of stilling the mind. If you have ever observed how fast your mind can race with thoughts, you will understand why people will say meditation is *hard*.

The mind is constantly bombarded with thoughts and the stress of our racing society exacerbates this human condition. When you can take your focus away from your thoughts during meditation and just be, you will discover an inner stillness.

Find a quiet place where you can sit comfortably. To ensure your spine is aligned properly, imagine yourself as a puppet with strings rising up through the crown of your head. Imagine the puppeteer pulling up on your strings and feel your spine lengthen.

Begin deep breathing.

Breathe in, breathe out. Breathe in, breathe out.

Allow your attention to remain on your breath in and your breath out. When thoughts cross your mind, see them as clouds passing by in the sky.

When you notice your attention on your thoughts, gently bring your awareness back to your breath.

That's all there is to it.

Meditation in nature is powerful. Allow your mind to be filled with the sounds of a gentle breeze or flowing water to drown out your racing mind.

Relaxing music is helpful as well. Emphasizing the sound of your breath can also fill the mind to make less room for intrusive thoughts.

Try starting with just two minutes every day and work up to twenty.

The more you practice, the easier this becomes. Thoughts will enter your mind more gently, you will be less distracted by their arrival and letting those thoughts go will come naturally.

As you master meditation, the quicker you are able to access your inner place of peace.

Anywhere. Anytime.

Calm in the chaos.

Step Four: Feel Deeply

Emotions are natural sensations that you experience as a human. How you react to an emotion creates a feeling. Feeling emotions is crucial to your wellbeing.

Letting go of emotions is uncomfortable and painful at times. Sometimes we hang onto them and these unexpressed emotions get buried deep inside.

The longer you hang onto what no longer serves you, the more painful it is when you *have* to let go.

When emotions come up, feel them deeply. Then let them go. Feel good about expressing yourself. Sigh. Relax into a sad day. Cry. Release your anger. Yell. Enjoy happiness and celebrate. Laugh and rejoice.

Once you get in tune with your feelings, these feelings can be used as a guide throughout life. When making decisions, you can choose what feels good and whether you are choosing between two different books to read, accepting a dinner invitation by a stranger, or choosing a new position at work, your feelings can help you make the best decision. What option makes you feel better?

Trust your gut.

Step Five: Express Gratitude

Giving thanks is great for your health. Gratitude is an attitude and a choice.

Keep a gratitude journal. Write down that for which you are grateful. Use details rather than just making a superficial list of things. You can include people, animals and how they touched your heart, as well as memorable moments, surprises and kind acts from the day.

Feel the depth of your gratitude in your heart. Make the conscious decision to be happier throughout the writing process.

Keeping a gratitude journal can be a very powerful habit. Whenever you are having an unpleasant day, take time to write in your journal. Allow gratitude to fill your heart and you will start feeling better.

If you want goodness to come into your life, it's important to appreciate what you already have.

Be grateful.

Step Six: Imagine

Create a vision board.

This can be a large cork board or a simple piece of paper. It is a space for visualization. Visualization is a powerful mind exercise.

Display your board in a place where you will see it often. Anything that inspires and motivates you can go onto your board such as magazine clippings, pictures, quotes and treasures from nature. Whatever you want to bring into your life, post it on your board. Add anything that makes you feel good.

But it's more than just thinking about things you want in your life. Make the focus of your board less about what you want and more about how you *feel*. If you want a new bike, how do you want that new bike to make you feel? Be sure your board reflects this feeling.

Make time everyday to look at your board and feel. Carry that feeling throughout your day.

Feelings are the key to being a master creator.

Live your dream.

Plan

Honeybees are a highly organized and complex society. Their hive is a super-organism. This means without all of the honeybees performing their individualized tasks, the hive would not survive.

No one gives orders, but everyone knows what to do. Good communication is the key.

Each bee has a series of jobs throughout its life to care for the colony; each duty is essential to the health of the hive.

When the hive is threatened, bees come together to defend it. When honeybees are sick, they leave the hive and sacrifice themselves for the wellbeing of the colony. When a deadly mite latches itself to a honeybee, other bees will try to pull it off. They help one another and work together.

Honey is the result of this teamwork.

Imagine a healthcare system where we worked together as well as honeybees in a hive.

Any individual who is motivated to live their best life is able to. A fair trade system ensures everyone has access to a caring community and compassionate care. People are provided wellness services in exchange for money, time, energy, and abilities. There is no discrimination.

All of us have something very unique to share with the world. Everyone has an important role like the honeybee in a colony.

People are encouraged to engage in sustainable living practices. They are given seeds, starts and cultures to begin cultivating their own food. Tending to and caring for the environment is learned through organic gardening, composting and rainwater collection.

Efforts are organized and there are a variety of community-oriented cooperatives such as sober, social grounds to support the military and Veterans and transitional housing for New Americans. There are establishments for trading trades, career development, and business coaching. We could have caring centers, which bring together seniors citizens and children. We could have organizations that connect lonely people with homeless animals.

In this society, there are housing projects where homeless people build their own self-sustainable housing and are provided the means to start living off the land. Veterans are given the education and tools to become small farmers for the local community or perhaps Vets use their new knowledge and skills to teach community members to do more of the same. Programs like these would encourage self-esteem, create purpose and grow community.

Each and every one of us has something to offer and contribute to the Greater Good.

All people and animals have their basic needs met and a healthy environment to thrive in: fresh air, clean water, nutritious food, a comfortable home, and loving support. The interconnectivity of all things is acknowledged and appreciated. Nature and Mother Earth is honored. Everything is tended to: the rivers, the oceans, the soil, plants, and trees.

Love, honor and respect for All is the standard.

How sweet would that be?

Genuine healthcare enhances the life of everyone and everything. Native Americans had a great understanding of spirit, community, and interconnectivity.

For them, becoming a warrior was a transformative process that started at a very young age. Elders knew the harsh realities of war and these were taught to the youngsters.

War was the last resort.

If battle was truly necessary for defending their people from real threat, warriors were sent into battle and the community mourned together.

When warriors returned, they were taken into the arms of the people. They were vulnerable with wounds deep, open, and tender and the community would tend to these physical, mental, emotional, and spiritual wounds. There were sacred ceremonies for all, including those who returned, those who didn't, and even those they fought and killed. All individuals in the community felt the trauma and pains of war. It was a healing process for *everyone*.

That is what healthcare should be like for Veterans.

Examination

Consider the hives that you are a member of.

• How do you contribute to the colony?

• How effective is your communication?

• Is there teamwork and togetherness?

• What is the health status of your hive?

• What are the fruits of your labor?

• What is threatening your hive?

• How can you create buzz about change?

• How does your hive contribute to the world?

Implementation

Take action!

Love yourself, listen to your body and respect your emotions. Tame your mind. Honor your divine self. Simplify and unclutter your life. Find purpose for your old stuff. Donate. See the good in everyone. Help people out. Drive less, walk and bike more. Practice yoga or Tai Chi. Spend more time in nature. Read inspirational books. Turn off the television programming and listen to news not owned by corporate interests. Focus on *good* things happening in the world. Listen to music that raises you up. Accept responsibility for your own happiness. Find your passion.

Follow your bliss. Trust the journey.

Be a conscious consumer. Eat organic and non-genetically modified foods. Take reusable bags to the grocery store. Switch to brands of companies that are socially responsible. Explore different health modalities. Get a certified health coach. See a naturopath. Go to a reflexologist. Experience a reiki master or other types of energy work. Use high quality, pure essential oils. For a diagnosis, get opinions from complementary practitioners. Keep your immune system strong. Eat cultured foods. Take a cooking class with your partner instead of eating out. Be aware of your socially accepted addictions. Hugs not drugs.

Let food be your medicine.

Raise the standards of care at the VA. Advocate for fair and just treatment of Veterans. Write your representatives. Encourage collaboration between Veterans, employees and community. Be concerned with the Veterans, not with the "numbers". Involve Vets in decision and policy making within the Veterans Administration. Let's listen to employee and Veteran suggestions locally and simplify VA processes. Teach effective communication skills to all employees from day one. Use the phonetic alphabet along with other practices familiar and second nature to Veterans. Welcome Veterans' planning and participation in facility events. Create a Veterans Association to influence and impact change in the VA. Be hospitable and open facilities to Veteran groups.

Be active in a worthy cause.

Let go of old ways of thinking and open yourselves up to new ideas. Educate yourself on the world's issues and be an informed citizen. Pay attention to politics. Be mindful of who you vote for. Step into leadership. Come up with logical solutions. Hold people accountable for their actions and attitudes. Fear not the ridicule and retaliation. Join forces with like-minded people. Stand up against tyranny. Question the cultural norm. Challenge yourself. Step out of your comfort zone even if it makes others uncomfortable, as well. Speak your truth. Be a voice for those without one. Inspire and involve others. Value life over money. Live your purpose.

Be the change and make a difference.

Case Study

It was six years ago that things really began to change in my life. The connection between my diet and lifestyle to my health became more obvious. The link between my everyday choices to the declining health of the planet was clear. I learned how food, emotions and environment were related to asthma and my breathing.

When I began exploring different health modalities, I was fascinated with all I could do naturally to breathe better. No longer was I going to "need" prescription medications.

I committed to change.

One step at a time, I began incorporating more healthful behaviors and replaced the not-so healthy habits. My home was rid of commercial cleaning products and switched to non-toxic agents like baking soda, vinegar, and essential oils. A Berkey water filter was purchased to cleanse drinking water of chemicals like chlorine. I dramatically decreased my consumption of meat and other animal products because of their devastating effect on the environment. I ate fewer foods with a package and more whole foods and transitioned to a colorful plant-based diet. I stopped using pharmaceutical drugs.

I was detoxing.

Everything about my health was improving.

I could take a full breath after years of not being able to breathe deeply. Weight dropped from my body. For the first time in years, my bowels were moving regularly with ease. My hair and nails became stronger. My skin was clear, my eyes were bright, and my teeth were even whiter.

I had more energy than I could ever remember and the more I detoxed, the clearer I was thinking.

It wasn't until the haze lifted did I recognize I'd been living with a serious anxiety disorder. I'd been cloudy for so long. By not putting as many chemicals and toxins in my body, my anxious thoughts were less frequent. The thoughts were still there, but they were less intrusive. Not being overrun by my worried mind allowed me to be present.

This changed everything.

Sleep was deep and uninterrupted. Sex was more pleasurable. Time management, attention to detail, and focus all improved. Work performance came easier. I was inspired to further my education and had the energy to do so.

Life was exponentially better.

As my mind settled, I was able to distinguish my thoughts from my intuition. I developed an intimate relationship with my spiritual self, discovering I am never alone and that I am always fully supported in this world.

When I was anxious, worried, overwhelmed or fearful, I would take a deep breath, ask for guidance, and trust my inner council.

As I became more aware, I learned how to tune into my feelings. These feelings became my internal compass for life. I let go of relationships that did not make me feel good; if a person made me feel uneasy, I used discretion. When making life decisions, I would choose that which made me feel better.

Everything was shifting.

For years I knew working for the VA was not supporting my wellbeing. My job made me feel more bad than good. Despite how bad working for the VA made me feel, letting go of a safe and secure job was very difficult. There were many excuses for keeping this job. The ones I used most often, I was serving those who served and getting paid to see the United States. In all honesty though, the most influential were related to my finances: no mortgage, a $60,000 salary and years invested in a federal retirement plan.

I was comfortable.

But I was not happy.

Anyone I told that I might leave the VA, reinforced my fears. They would say, "What will you do for health benefits?" "What is your plan for retirement?" "Won't you miss all the paid federal holidays?" My unsatisfied and uninspired coworkers were more concerned about my paycheck than my passion but I knew what I had to do.

Do what you love and love what you do.
Money and abundance will follow.

I abruptly resigned from the VA and began writing this book. The transition from federal employee and travel nurse to author and holistic entrepreneur has been uncomfortable at times. Despite the discomfort, I couldn't be happier with my decision.

I am doing what I love and feeling really good about it. I have the energy to follow my dreams and trusting in my vision.

Hive Life Enhancement.

Hive Life Enhancement provides simple and effective wellness education, nutritional guidance, action accountability, and energy enhancement for people who are ready, willing, and able, particularly, healthcare professionals. Our mission is to be a catalyst for positive and progressive change in the healthcare delivery system. Healthcare professionals must be well themselves for them be effective in their professional roles.

Inspired by nature and the bees, Hive Life Enhancement focuses on caring relationships with yourself, fellow humans beings, all animals, and the environment.

Hive Life Enhancement has a pharmaceutical-free approach to wellness that empowers and energizes individuals to optimize their quality of life. We can help you transition off of pharmaceutical drugs, processed foods, and sugar, and teach you how to truly nourish your mind, body, and soul.

Hive Life Enhancement is building the foundation of an online wellness platform for Veterans. Our hope is that we'll have such a significant impact on Veterans' wellbeing that physical chapters, or "Hives", will be established nationwide. This community would be similar to an organization like the VFW but with a focus on Veterans' health and sustainable living practices. My intention for this community is to uphold the values of an honest and effective healthcare system.

- Awareness.
- Accountability.
- Communication.
- Collaboration.
- Teamwork.
- Togetherness.

Change

There is no simple solution to the healthcare crisis. It's complex and extends far beyond our nation's borders. What we are doing to patients is what we are doing to the planet.

This is a global health crisis. The messages are becoming harder to ignore. Our systems have to change and so do we.

Change is so intimidating that people will deny the need to change for years. People will ignore physical and emotional pain until it becomes unbearable. The thought of change is often so overwhelming that most people just continue doing what they've always done. Perfectionism and fear of failure prevent people from taking action. Many know what they need to do for their health but don't know how to accomplish it.

This is similiar to how people react to community, organizational, and global issues.

People fear change and discomfort. "How will my life be different?"

People are afraid to stand up and speak out. "What will happen if I do?"

People feel powerless. "What difference do I make?"

Knowing that there is an issue, but not knowing what to do next can be paralyzing.

If you want things in your life to change, you start by acknowledging the need to change and then take the first step. No matter how big or small, any positive change in your life matters. Commit. Keep moving forward. The path isn't always smooth and missteps will happen. Just keep going. As you shift, grow, and evolve, you gain momentum. You become unstoppable.

The same thing happens with the world. And it's happening right now. Grassroots movements of all kinds are starting everywhere. People are stepping into their power. They are dreaming big, following their hearts and believing. These people are changing the world.

Transformative change is happening and its not slowing down. Momentum is building. You can be a part of this grassroots revolution. We need you to be part of this. Everyone of us has a role in making this a better world.

We are *all* part of the solution.

<u>Conclusion</u>

Cultural beliefs and values are so deeply rooted into our being that they are rarely questioned. When a cultural change is necessary, many do not see the need. They are just doing what has always been done.

Most people know of no other way, nor do they even consider that there *is* another way. People just do what they know. These people do what everyone does, because that's what everyone is doing.

Others may question the norm but change is viewed as impossible and they expend little energy in creating a solution. As awful as it may be, "it's just the way it is" and "it'll never change." These people keep moving along with the herd.

However, more and more people are realizing we are living in a broken system and are looking for a new way, but they don't know what to do or how to do it.

The world needs brave people, strong leaders and dedicated followers to be the change. When everyday people, like you and I, value life over money, take care of eachother, and love ourselves and one another, we create a culture of caring. We create that possibility for people.

We show people the way.

Resources

Books:

Awakening to the Spirit World: The Shamanic Path of Direct Revelation. Ingerman, S., & Wesselman, H. (2010).

The Book of Understanding: Creating Your Own Path to Freedom. Osho (2006).

E-Squared: Nine Do-It-Yourself Energy Experiments That Prove Your Thoughts Create Your Reality. Grout, P. (2012).

The Food Revolution: How Your Diet Can Help Save Your Life and Our World. Robbins, J. (2001).

Green Medicine: Challenging the Assumptions of Conventional Health Care. Malerba, L. (2010).

The Untethered Soul: A Journey Beyond Yourself. Singer, M. (2007).

War and The Soul: Healing Our Nation's Veterans from Post-traumatic Stress Disorder. Tick, E. (2005).

Warrior's Return: Restoring the Soul After War. Tick, E. (2014).

Causes:

Soldier's Heart (soldiersheart.net)

Weed For Warriors Project (wfwproject.org)

Documentaries:

Fed Up. (Soechtig, 2014) Film.

I Am. (Shadyac, 2012) Film.

Cowspiracy: The Sustainability Secret. (Anderson & Kuhn, 2015) Film.

Inspiration and News:

Hay House Radio (hayhouseradio.com)

National Public Radio (npr.org)

The Optimist Magazine (theoptimist.com)

Yes! Magazine (yesmagazine.org)

The Young Turks (tytnetwork.com)

Music:

Nahko and Medicine for the People

Rising Appalachia

About the Author

From certified nursing assistant to registered nurse, Erin has spent thirteen years in the healthcare system. She traveled throughout the United States and toured six different VA facilities in various nursing roles. With a passion for health education and empowerment, Erin became an Integrative Nutrition health coach and a certified Trailblazing Communications practitioner. Erin founded Hive Life Enhancement and provides wellness education, nutritional guidance, action accountability and energy enhancement to Veterans across the nation. She's a dancing queen who appreciates authentic musicians and soulful music. Erin enjoys outdoor adventures and spending time in nature. For now, Moorhead, Minnesota is her home.

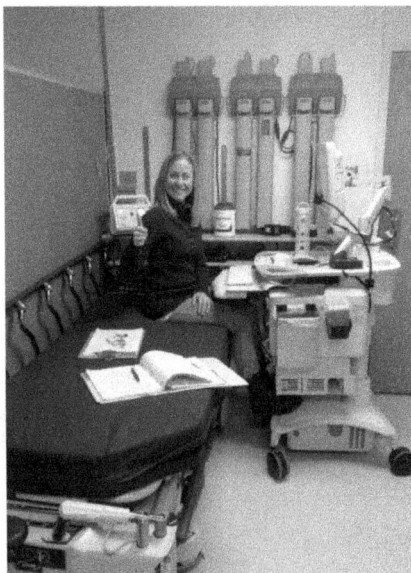

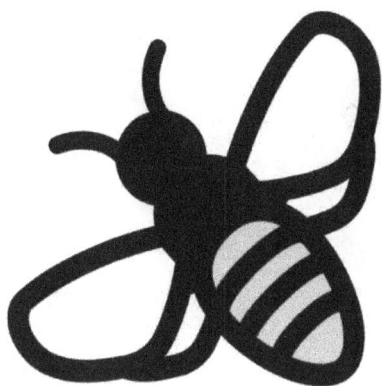